Chapter 1: Understanding the Prostate Gland

The Anatomy of the Prostate Gland

The prostate gland is a small, walnut-sized organ located below the bladder in men. It plays a crucial role in the reproductive system by producing seminal fluid, which helps transport sperm during ejaculation. Understanding the anatomy of the prostate gland is essential for maintaining good prostate health and preventing potential issues.

The prostate gland is made up of several different types of tissue, including glandular tissue, muscle tissue, and fibrous tissue. The glandular tissue is responsible for producing the fluid that makes up the majority of semen. The muscle tissue helps the prostate contract during ejaculation, while the fibrous tissue provides structural support to the gland.

One of the key components of the prostate gland is the prostate-specific antigen (PSA), a protein produced by the gland. PSA levels can be measured through a blood test and are used as a marker for potential prostate issues such as inflammation, infection, or cancer. Monitoring PSA levels regularly is important for detecting any abnormalities early on.

The prostate gland is surrounded by a network of nerves and blood vessels that are vital for its function. These nerves and blood vessels are responsible for controlling the flow of blood to the prostate, as well as transmitting signals between the brain and the gland. Damage to these structures can result in issues such as erectile dysfunction or urinary problems.

In conclusion, understanding the anatomy of the prostate gland is crucial for maintaining good prostate health. By knowing how the gland functions and what structures are involved, men can take proactive steps to prevent potential issues and maintain optimal prostate function. Regular check-ups, monitoring PSA levels, and leading a healthy lifestyle are all important factors in promoting prostate health and overall well-being.

Function of the Prostate Gland

The prostate gland is a vital component of the male reproductive system, responsible for producing a fluid that helps nourish and transport sperm. Located just below the bladder and in front of the rectum, the prostate gland is a small, walnut-sized organ that plays a crucial role in a man's overall health. Understanding the function of the prostate gland is essential for maintaining optimal prostate health.

One of the primary functions of the prostate gland is to produce prostate-specific antigen (PSA), a protein that helps liquefy semen and aids in sperm mobility. PSA levels can be an indicator of prostate health, with elevated levels potentially signaling prostate issues such as inflammation, infection, or even cancer. Regular prostate screenings, including PSA tests, are recommended for men over the age of 50 to monitor prostate health and detect any potential issues early on.

In addition to producing PSA, the prostate gland also plays a role in controlling urine flow. The prostate surrounds the urethra, the tube that carries urine from the bladder out of the body. As the prostate gland grows larger with age, it can put pressure on the urethra, leading to urinary symptoms such as frequent urination, weak urine stream, and difficulty emptying the bladder. This condition, known as benign prostatic hyperplasia (BPH), is common among older men and can impact quality of life if left untreated.

Maintaining a healthy prostate gland is crucial for overall well-being. A balanced diet rich in fruits, vegetables, and whole grains, along with regular exercise, can help reduce the risk of prostate issues. Avoiding tobacco and excessive alcohol consumption, as well as maintaining a healthy weight, can also contribute to prostate health. Additionally, staying hydrated and practicing good hygiene can help prevent urinary tract infections that may affect the prostate gland.

In conclusion, the prostate gland plays a vital role in male reproductive and urinary health. Understanding its functions and taking proactive steps to maintain prostate health is essential for every man. By staying informed, adopting healthy lifestyle habits, and scheduling regular prostate screenings, men can reduce their risk of developing prostate issues and ensure optimal prostate health for years to come.

Common Prostate Health Issues

Prostate health is a topic that is often overlooked by many men, but it is crucial to understand the common issues that can arise in this area of the body. One of the most common prostate health issues is benign prostatic hyperplasia (BPH), which is a non-cancerous enlargement of the prostate gland. This condition can cause symptoms such as frequent urination, difficulty starting or maintaining a stream of urine, and a feeling of incomplete emptying of the bladder.

Another common prostate health issue is prostatitis, which is inflammation of the prostate gland. This condition can be acute or chronic and can cause symptoms such as pain in the pelvic area, difficulty urinating, and pain during ejaculation. Prostatitis can be caused by bacterial infections, but in some cases, the cause is unknown.

Prostate cancer is another common prostate health issue that men should be aware of. Prostate cancer is the most common cancer in men, and it is estimated that one in nine men will be diagnosed with the disease in their lifetime. Symptoms of prostate cancer can include difficulty urinating, blood in the urine or semen, and pain in the back, hips, or pelvis. Early detection and treatment of prostate cancer are crucial for a successful outcome.

Other common prostate health issues include erectile dysfunction, which can be a result of prostate surgery or other treatments for prostate conditions. Erectile dysfunction can have a significant impact on a man's quality of life and self-esteem. Incontinence is another common issue that can arise after prostate surgery or as a result of other prostate conditions. It is important for men to seek help from a healthcare provider if they are experiencing any of these symptoms or issues related to their prostate health.

In conclusion, understanding the common prostate health issues that men may face is essential for maintaining overall health and well-being. By being aware of the symptoms and risk factors associated with prostate conditions, men can take proactive steps to protect their prostate health and seek appropriate medical care when needed. Regular check-ups with a healthcare provider and maintaining a healthy lifestyle can help prevent and manage many prostate health issues. Remember, knowledge is power when it comes to your prostate health.

Chapter 2: Symptoms of Prostate Problems

Early Warning Signs

As men age, it is important to pay attention to the early warning signs of prostate health issues. Prostate problems can develop slowly over time, often without any noticeable symptoms. However, there are certain signs that should not be ignored. Knowing what to look for can help you catch potential issues early and seek proper treatment before they escalate.

One of the most common early warning signs of prostate issues is difficulty urinating. This can manifest as a weak or interrupted urine flow, frequent urination (especially at night), or a feeling of urgency that you need to urinate right away. If you are experiencing any of these symptoms, it is important to consult with your healthcare provider to determine the underlying cause.

Another early warning sign of prostate problems is pain or discomfort in the pelvic area, lower back, or hips. This may be a sign of inflammation or infection in the prostate gland. In some cases, you may also experience pain during ejaculation or blood in the semen. These symptoms should not be ignored and should be evaluated by a healthcare professional.

Changes in sexual function can also be an early warning sign of prostate health issues. This may include erectile dysfunction, decreased libido, or difficulty achieving or maintaining an erection. While these symptoms can have various causes, they can also be linked to prostate problems. It is important to discuss any changes in sexual function with your doctor to determine the best course of action.

In conclusion, being aware of the early warning signs of prostate health issues is crucial for maintaining optimal health as a man. By paying attention to symptoms such as difficulty urinating, pelvic pain, and changes in sexual function, you can catch potential problems early and seek appropriate treatment. Remember, early detection and intervention can make a significant difference in your prostate health outcomes. Don't hesitate to consult with your healthcare provider if you are experiencing any concerning symptoms.

Advanced Symptoms

In this subchapter, we will delve into the advanced symptoms of prostate health issues that every man should be aware of. It is crucial to understand that while some symptoms may be common, others may indicate more serious underlying conditions. By recognizing these advanced symptoms, you can take proactive steps to address any potential issues and maintain optimal prostate health.

One of the advanced symptoms to be mindful of is persistent urinary problems. This may include increased frequency of urination, difficulty starting or stopping urination, or a weak urine flow. These symptoms can be indicative of conditions such as benign prostatic hyperplasia (BPH) or even prostate cancer. If you experience any of these symptoms, it is important to consult with your healthcare provider for a thorough evaluation.

Another advanced symptom to watch out for is blood in the urine or semen. While this may be alarming, it is not always a cause for immediate concern. However, it is essential to rule out more serious conditions such as prostate cancer. If you notice any abnormal bleeding, it is crucial to seek medical attention promptly for further evaluation and diagnosis.

Additionally, persistent pain in the pelvic area, lower back, or hips can be a sign of advanced prostate health issues. This discomfort may be a result of inflammation, infection, or even the presence of prostate cancer. If you experience ongoing pain in these areas, it is essential to speak with your healthcare provider to determine the underlying cause and appropriate treatment options.

In conclusion, being vigilant about advanced symptoms of prostate health issues is crucial for maintaining overall well-being. By staying informed and proactive, you can take control of your health and address any potential concerns early on. Remember, early detection and treatment are key to managing prostate health conditions effectively. Do not hesitate to seek medical advice if you notice any advanced symptoms or changes in your prostate health.

When to See a Doctor

When it comes to prostate health, it is important to know when to seek medical attention. While it is normal for men to experience some symptoms related to their prostate as they age, there are certain signs that should not be ignored. If you are experiencing frequent urination, especially at night, or have difficulty starting or stopping urination, it may be time to see a doctor. These symptoms could indicate an enlarged prostate or even prostate cancer, so it is important to get checked out as soon as possible.

Another reason to see a doctor regarding prostate health is if you are experiencing pain or discomfort in your pelvic area. This could be a sign of prostatitis, which is an inflammation of the prostate gland. Prostatitis can be caused by a bacterial infection or other factors, and it is important to get it treated promptly to prevent further complications. Your doctor can perform tests to determine the cause of your symptoms and recommend appropriate treatment options.

If you notice blood in your urine or semen, it is crucial to see a doctor right away. These symptoms could be a sign of prostate cancer, which is the second most common cancer in men. Early detection is key to successful treatment, so do not hesitate to seek medical attention if you notice any unusual changes in your urine or semen. Your doctor can perform tests such as a prostate-specific antigen (PSA) test or a biopsy to determine if cancer is present.

In addition to physical symptoms, changes in your sexual function can also indicate a problem with your prostate. If you are experiencing erectile dysfunction, painful ejaculation, or a decrease in libido, it may be related to prostate health issues. These symptoms could be caused by an enlarged prostate, prostatitis, or even prostate cancer. Seeing a doctor can help determine the underlying cause of your sexual health changes and provide appropriate treatment options.

Overall, it is important for men to pay attention to their prostate health and seek medical attention if they notice any concerning symptoms. Regular check-ups with a healthcare provider can help catch potential issues early and prevent serious complications down the line. Remember, your health is important, so do not hesitate to see a doctor if you have any concerns about your prostate health.

Chapter 3: Prostate Health Screening

Importance of Regular Check-ups

Regular check-ups are essential for maintaining good prostate health. By scheduling routine visits with your healthcare provider, you can catch any potential issues early on and take steps to prevent more serious problems down the line. Prostate cancer, one of the most common cancers in men, often shows no symptoms in its early stages. Regular check-ups can help detect prostate cancer early when it is most treatable.

In addition to catching potential issues early, regular check-ups also allow your healthcare provider to monitor your overall prostate health and make recommendations for preventative measures. By keeping track of your prostate health over time, your healthcare provider can identify any changes or abnormalities that may require further investigation. This proactive approach can help you stay ahead of any potential problems and take action to maintain optimal prostate health.

Furthermore, regular check-ups can help you stay informed about the latest developments in prostate health and treatment options. Your healthcare provider can provide you with up-to-date information on screening guidelines, lifestyle changes, and treatment options that may be relevant to your individual health needs. By staying informed and proactive about your prostate health, you can make informed decisions about your care and take steps to protect yourself from potential risks.

Regular check-ups also provide an opportunity for open communication with your healthcare provider about any concerns or questions you may have regarding your prostate health. By building a strong relationship with your healthcare provider, you can feel comfortable discussing sensitive topics and seeking guidance on how to best care for your prostate. This open dialogue can empower you to take control of your health and make informed decisions about your prostate care.

In conclusion, regular check-ups are a crucial aspect of maintaining good prostate health. By scheduling routine visits with your healthcare provider, you can catch potential issues early, monitor your prostate health over time, stay informed about the latest developments in prostate health, and build a strong relationship with your healthcare provider. Taking a proactive approach to your prostate health through regular check-ups can help you stay ahead of any potential problems and take steps to protect yourself from risks. Remember, your health is your greatest asset – prioritize it by scheduling regular check-ups today.

Types of Screening Tests

When it comes to maintaining optimal prostate health, one important aspect to consider is undergoing regular screening tests. Screening tests are essential in detecting any potential issues early on, allowing for timely intervention and treatment. There are several types of screening tests available for assessing prostate health, each serving a specific purpose in evaluating the condition of the prostate gland.

The first type of screening test is the Prostate-Specific Antigen (PSA) test. This blood test measures the levels of PSA in the blood, which is a protein produced by the prostate gland. Elevated levels of PSA can indicate a potential issue with the prostate, such as inflammation or enlargement. While a high PSA level does not necessarily mean prostate cancer, it is an important marker that warrants further investigation.

Another common screening test is the digital rectal exam (DRE), which involves a healthcare provider inserting a gloved, lubricated finger into the rectum to feel the prostate gland for any abnormalities. The DRE allows for a physical examination of the prostate gland, checking for any lumps, bumps, or changes in size or texture. This test is often performed in conjunction with the PSA test to provide a more comprehensive assessment of prostate health.

Imaging tests, such as ultrasound or MRI scans, may also be used as screening tests for prostate health. These tests provide detailed images of the prostate gland, allowing healthcare providers to visualize any abnormalities or changes in the structure of the gland. Imaging tests are often recommended if other screening tests indicate a potential issue with the prostate gland, or if further evaluation is needed to determine the cause of symptoms.

Genetic testing is another type of screening test that may be recommended for men with a family history of prostate cancer. Genetic testing can identify specific gene mutations that increase the risk of developing prostate cancer, allowing for personalized screening and prevention strategies. By identifying genetic risk factors early on, men can take proactive steps to monitor their prostate health and reduce their risk of developing prostate cancer.

In conclusion, there are several types of screening tests available for assessing prostate health, each serving a specific purpose in evaluating the condition of the prostate gland. From the PSA test to the DRE and imaging tests, these screening tests play a crucial role in detecting potential issues early on and guiding appropriate treatment and management strategies. Men should work closely with their healthcare providers to determine the most appropriate screening tests based on their individual risk factors, family history, and overall health status. Regular screening tests are essential for maintaining optimal prostate health and reducing the risk of developing prostate cancer.

Understanding PSA Levels

Prostate-specific antigen (PSA) levels are an important indicator of prostate health that every man should be aware of. PSA is a protein produced by the cells of the prostate gland and is typically found in small amounts in the blood. Elevated PSA levels can be a sign of various prostate conditions, including prostate cancer, prostatitis, and benign prostatic hyperplasia (BPH). Monitoring PSA levels regularly can help detect potential issues early and guide appropriate treatment decisions.

It is important to understand that PSA levels can fluctuate for a variety of reasons. Age, race, family history, and certain medications can all impact PSA levels. It is also normal for PSA levels to increase slightly with age, so it is essential to establish a baseline PSA level and monitor changes over time. If PSA levels are found to be elevated, further testing may be needed to determine the cause and appropriate course of action.

When interpreting PSA levels, it is crucial to consider the context of the individual patient. A high PSA level does not necessarily mean a man has prostate cancer, as other factors such as inflammation or infection can also cause elevated PSA levels. Conversely, a low PSA level does not guarantee that a man is free from prostate cancer. It is important to discuss PSA levels with a healthcare provider who can provide personalized guidance based on the individual's risk factors and overall health.

Regular screenings for PSA levels are recommended for men over the age of 50, or earlier for those with a family history of prostate cancer or other risk factors. Screening frequency may vary based on individual risk factors and should be discussed with a healthcare provider. Understanding PSA levels and their implications is an essential part of maintaining prostate health and overall well-being. By staying informed and proactive about prostate health, men can take control of their health and make informed decisions about their care.

Chapter 4: Lifestyle Factors for Prostate Health

Diet and Nutrition

Diet and nutrition play a crucial role in maintaining prostate health. Making healthy food choices can help reduce the risk of prostate problems and promote overall well-being. In this subchapter, we will explore the impact of diet on prostate health and provide practical tips for incorporating a prostate-friendly diet into your daily routine.

Research has shown that certain foods can have a positive effect on prostate health. Foods rich in antioxidants, such as fruits and vegetables, can help reduce inflammation and oxidative stress in the body. This, in turn, may lower the risk of developing prostate cancer and other prostate-related issues. Including a variety of colorful fruits and vegetables in your diet can provide a range of vitamins, minerals, and phytochemicals that support prostate health.

In addition to fruits and vegetables, incorporating healthy fats into your diet is important for prostate health. Omega-3 fatty acids, found in fatty fish like salmon and walnuts, have anti-inflammatory properties that may help protect the prostate. Limiting saturated and trans fats, which are often found in processed foods and red meat, can also help reduce inflammation and support prostate health.

It is also important to pay attention to your overall calorie intake and maintain a healthy weight. Being overweight or obese has been linked to an increased risk of developing prostate cancer and other prostate-related issues. By following a balanced diet that includes a variety of nutrient-dense foods and practicing portion control, you can help manage your weight and support your prostate health.

In conclusion, making smart choices about what you eat can have a significant impact on your prostate health. By focusing on a diet rich in fruits, vegetables, healthy fats, and lean proteins, you can lower your risk of developing prostate problems and promote overall well-being. Remember to consult with your healthcare provider or a registered dietitian for personalized nutrition advice tailored to your specific needs and goals.

Exercise and Physical Activity

Exercise and physical activity play a crucial role in maintaining prostate health. Regular exercise has been shown to reduce the risk of developing prostate cancer, as well as promoting overall prostate health. Men who engage in regular physical activity are less likely to experience symptoms of prostate enlargement or inflammation. Additionally, exercise can help improve circulation to the prostate gland, which can aid in preventing the development of prostate-related issues.

One of the key benefits of exercise for prostate health is its ability to reduce inflammation in the body. Chronic inflammation has been linked to an increased risk of developing prostate cancer, so incorporating regular exercise into your routine can help lower this risk. Exercise also helps to regulate hormone levels, which can further contribute to a healthy prostate. By maintaining a healthy weight through exercise, men can also reduce their risk of developing prostate issues, as obesity has been linked to an increased risk of prostate cancer.

In addition to reducing the risk of prostate cancer, exercise can also help manage symptoms of prostate enlargement, also known as benign prostatic hyperplasia (BPH). Regular physical activity can help improve urinary flow and reduce the frequency of nighttime urination, which are common symptoms of BPH. By strengthening the pelvic floor muscles through exercise, men can also improve bladder control and reduce the risk of urinary incontinence.

It's important for men to incorporate a variety of exercises into their routine to promote optimal prostate health. Aerobic exercises, such as running, swimming, or cycling, can help improve cardiovascular health and circulation to the prostate gland. Strength training exercises, such as weightlifting or bodyweight exercises, can help build muscle mass and improve overall physical fitness. Additionally, incorporating flexibility exercises, such as yoga or stretching, can help improve range of motion and prevent injury during physical activity.

In conclusion, exercise and physical activity are essential components of maintaining prostate health. By incorporating regular exercise into your routine, you can reduce your risk of developing prostate cancer, manage symptoms of prostate enlargement, and improve overall prostate health. Remember to consult with your healthcare provider before starting any new exercise program, especially if you have existing prostate issues. With a commitment to regular physical activity, you can take proactive steps towards promoting a healthy prostate and overall well-being.

Stress Management and Mental Health

Stress Management and Mental Health are crucial components of maintaining overall prostate health. Stress has been shown to have a negative impact on the body, including the prostate gland. When stress levels are high, the body releases cortisol, a hormone that can suppress the immune system and increase inflammation. This can lead to a variety of health issues, including prostate problems. Therefore, it is important for men to prioritize stress management techniques in order to protect their prostate health.

One of the most effective ways to manage stress is through relaxation techniques such as deep breathing, meditation, and yoga. These practices can help to calm the mind and reduce the body's stress response. Additionally, regular exercise has been shown to be beneficial for both mental health and prostate health. Exercise releases endorphins, which are natural mood lifters, and can help to reduce stress levels.

In addition to relaxation techniques and exercise, it is important for men to prioritize self-care and make time for activities that bring them joy and relaxation. This can include hobbies, spending time with loved ones, and engaging in activities that promote mental well-being. By taking time for themselves and practicing self-care, men can reduce their stress levels and improve their overall mental health.

It is also important for men to seek professional help if they are struggling with stress or mental health issues. Talking to a therapist or counselor can provide valuable tools and strategies for managing stress and improving mental well-being. Additionally, medication or other treatments may be necessary for some men to effectively manage their mental health.

By prioritizing stress management and mental health, men can take proactive steps to protect their prostate health and overall well-being. By incorporating relaxation techniques, exercise, self-care, and seeking professional help when needed, men can reduce their stress levels and improve their mental health, leading to a healthier prostate and a higher quality of life.

Chapter 5: Natural Remedies for Prostate Health

Herbal Supplements

Herbal supplements have become increasingly popular in recent years as men seek alternative methods to support their prostate health. While not a cure-all, many herbal supplements have shown promise in helping to maintain prostate health and reduce the risk of developing prostate issues. It is important for men to understand the potential benefits and risks associated with herbal supplements before incorporating them into their daily routine.

One of the most well-known herbal supplements for prostate health is saw palmetto. This plant extract has been used for centuries to support urinary and prostate health. Research has shown that saw palmetto may help reduce the symptoms of an enlarged prostate, such as frequent urination and difficulty starting urination. However, it is important to consult with a healthcare provider before starting any new supplement regimen, as saw palmetto may interact with certain medications.

Another popular herbal supplement for prostate health is beta-sitosterol. This plant sterol is found in many fruits, vegetables, nuts, and seeds, and has been shown to help reduce inflammation in the prostate gland. Beta-sitosterol may also help improve urinary flow and reduce the risk of developing prostate issues. As with any supplement, it is important to carefully read the label and follow the recommended dosage guidelines.

Pygeum is another herbal supplement that has been used for centuries to support prostate health. This plant extract has been shown to help reduce inflammation in the prostate gland and improve urinary flow. Pygeum may also help reduce the risk of developing prostate issues, such as benign prostatic hyperplasia (BPH). Men interested in incorporating pygeum into their daily routine should consult with a healthcare provider to ensure it is safe and appropriate for their individual health needs.

In conclusion, herbal supplements can be a valuable addition to a man's prostate health regimen. However, it is important to approach these supplements with caution and consult with a healthcare provider before starting any new regimen. By understanding the potential benefits and risks associated with herbal supplements, men can make informed decisions about how to support their prostate health and overall well-being.

Essential Nutrients

In order to maintain optimal prostate health, it is essential for men to ensure they are consuming the necessary nutrients that support the function of this vital organ. Essential nutrients play a crucial role in preventing prostate issues such as inflammation, enlargement, and even cancer. By incorporating a balanced diet rich in these nutrients, men can significantly reduce their risk of developing prostate problems and promote overall well-being.

One of the key nutrients that men should prioritize for prostate health is zinc. Zinc plays a crucial role in maintaining prostate function and has been shown to help reduce the risk of prostate cancer. Foods such as oysters, beef, and pumpkin seeds are excellent sources of zinc and should be included in a man's diet on a regular basis. Additionally, selenium is another essential nutrient that has been linked to a lower risk of prostate cancer. Men can find selenium in foods like Brazil nuts, tuna, and sunflower seeds.

Omega-3 fatty acids are another important nutrient for prostate health. These healthy fats have anti-inflammatory properties that can help reduce inflammation in the prostate and lower the risk of developing prostate cancer. Foods such as fatty fish, flaxseeds, and walnuts are rich sources of omega-3 fatty acids and should be included in a man's diet regularly. In addition, lycopene, a powerful antioxidant found in tomatoes, has been shown to have protective effects on the prostate. Men should aim to consume foods high in lycopene, such as cooked tomatoes, tomato sauce, and watermelon, to support prostate health.

Vitamin D is another essential nutrient that plays a crucial role in prostate health. Studies have shown that men with low levels of vitamin D are at a higher risk of developing prostate cancer. To ensure optimal levels of vitamin D, men should spend time outdoors in the sun, as well as consume foods like fatty fish, egg yolks, and fortified dairy products. In addition to these nutrients, a diet rich in fruits, vegetables, whole grains, and lean proteins can provide the essential vitamins and minerals needed to support overall prostate health.

In conclusion, by prioritizing essential nutrients in their diet, men can take proactive steps to support their prostate health and reduce the risk of developing prostate issues. Zinc, selenium, omega-3 fatty acids, lycopene, and vitamin D are just a few of the key nutrients that men should focus on incorporating into their daily meals. By maintaining a balanced diet that includes a variety of nutrient-rich foods, men can promote optimal prostate function and overall well-being. Remember, a healthy diet is a key component of prostate health and should be a top priority for men looking to protect this vital organ.

Lifestyle Changes

Lifestyle changes play a crucial role in maintaining optimal prostate health. As men, it is important to be mindful of our habits and make necessary adjustments to promote a healthy prostate. By incorporating simple yet effective changes into our daily routine, we can reduce the risk of developing prostate issues and improve overall well-being.

One of the key lifestyle changes that can benefit prostate health is maintaining a healthy diet. Consuming a diet rich in fruits, vegetables, whole grains, and lean proteins can provide essential nutrients that support prostate function. Limiting the intake of red meat, processed foods, and sugary beverages is also important, as these items have been linked to an increased risk of prostate problems.

Regular exercise is another vital component of a healthy lifestyle that can positively impact prostate health. Engaging in physical activity on a regular basis can help reduce inflammation, improve circulation, and support overall prostate function. Aim for at least 30 minutes of moderate exercise most days of the week, such as walking, jogging, or cycling, to reap the benefits for your prostate.

Managing stress levels is also essential for maintaining a healthy prostate. Chronic stress can have a negative impact on prostate health, as it can lead to hormonal imbalances and increased inflammation. Finding healthy ways to cope with stress, such as exercise, meditation, or spending time in nature, can help protect your prostate and improve your overall quality of life.

In conclusion, making simple lifestyle changes can have a significant impact on prostate health. By focusing on maintaining a healthy diet, engaging in regular exercise, and managing stress levels, men can support their prostate function and reduce the risk of developing prostate problems. It is never too late to make positive changes that can benefit your prostate health and overall well-being.

Chapter 6: Medical Treatments for Prostate Conditions

Medications

Medications play a crucial role in the management of prostate health issues. There are several types of medications that are commonly prescribed to men with prostate conditions, such as benign prostatic hyperplasia (BPH) or prostate cancer. These medications can help alleviate symptoms, slow disease progression, and improve quality of life for those affected by prostate issues.

One common class of medications used in the treatment of BPH is alpha blockers. These medications work by relaxing the muscles in the prostate and bladder, which can help reduce urinary symptoms such as frequent urination, hesitancy, and weak urine stream. Alpha blockers are often prescribed as a first-line treatment for BPH and can provide relief for many men with this condition.

Another type of medication commonly used to treat BPH is 5-alpha reductase inhibitors. These medications work by reducing the levels of dihydrotestosterone (DHT), a hormone that contributes to prostate enlargement. By lowering DHT levels, 5-alpha reductase inhibitors can help shrink the prostate gland and improve urinary symptoms in men with BPH.

For men with prostate cancer, medications such as hormone therapy may be prescribed. Hormone therapy works by reducing the levels of testosterone in the body, which can help slow the growth of prostate cancer cells. This type of medication is often used in combination with other treatments, such as surgery or radiation therapy, to effectively manage prostate cancer and improve outcomes for patients.

It is important for men with prostate health issues to work closely with their healthcare providers to determine the most appropriate medication regimen for their specific condition. It is also important to follow the prescribed treatment plan and attend regular follow-up appointments to monitor the effectiveness of the medications and make any necessary adjustments. By taking an active role in their healthcare and working with their healthcare team, men can effectively manage their prostate health and improve their overall quality of life.

Surgical Procedures

Surgical procedures are often considered as a last resort in the treatment of prostate health issues. However, in certain cases, surgery may be necessary to address conditions such as prostate cancer or benign prostatic hyperplasia (BPH). It is important for men to understand the different types of surgical procedures available and the potential risks and benefits associated with each option.

One common surgical procedure for treating prostate cancer is radical prostatectomy, which involves the removal of the entire prostate gland. This procedure is typically recommended for men with localized prostate cancer that has not spread beyond the prostate gland. While radical prostatectomy can be effective in removing the cancerous tissue, it may also result in side effects such as urinary incontinence and erectile dysfunction.

Another surgical procedure that may be used to treat prostate cancer is radiation therapy. This treatment involves using high-energy rays to target and destroy cancer cells in the prostate gland. Radiation therapy may be used alone or in combination with other treatments such as surgery or hormone therapy. While radiation therapy can be effective in treating prostate cancer, it may also cause side effects such as fatigue, skin irritation, and urinary problems.

For men with benign prostatic hyperplasia (BPH), transurethral resection of the prostate (TURP) is a common surgical procedure used to relieve symptoms such as urinary frequency, urgency, and weak urine flow. During a TURP procedure, a surgeon uses a special instrument to remove excess tissue from the prostate gland, thereby improving urinary function. While TURP can be effective in relieving symptoms of BPH, it may also result in side effects such as retrograde ejaculation and urinary incontinence.

In conclusion, surgical procedures play an important role in the treatment of prostate health issues such as prostate cancer and benign prostatic hyperplasia. It is crucial for men to discuss their treatment options with a healthcare provider to determine the most appropriate course of action based on their individual circumstances. While surgery may come with potential risks and side effects, it can also offer significant benefits in terms of improving quality of life and overall health. Men should be proactive in educating themselves about surgical procedures and actively participate in the decision-making process regarding their prostate health.

Radiation Therapy

Radiation therapy is a commonly used treatment option for prostate cancer, offering men an effective way to target and eliminate cancerous cells in the prostate gland. This non-invasive procedure involves the use of high-energy radiation beams to destroy cancer cells and prevent them from multiplying. Radiation therapy can be used as a primary treatment for localized prostate cancer or as an adjuvant therapy following surgery to remove the prostate.

There are two main types of radiation therapy used to treat prostate cancer: external beam radiation therapy and brachytherapy. External beam radiation therapy involves delivering radiation from a machine outside the body to the prostate gland. This treatment is typically administered over a period of several weeks, with daily sessions lasting only a few minutes each. Brachytherapy, on the other hand, involves implanting radioactive seeds directly into the prostate gland to deliver targeted radiation therapy over a period of weeks or months.

One of the key advantages of radiation therapy for prostate cancer is its ability to target cancer cells while minimizing damage to surrounding healthy tissue. This precision helps to reduce the risk of side effects and complications commonly associated with other treatment options, such as surgery. Radiation therapy can also be used in combination with other treatments, such as hormone therapy, to improve outcomes for men with more advanced prostate cancer.

It is important for men considering radiation therapy for prostate cancer to discuss the potential risks and benefits with their healthcare provider. While radiation therapy is generally well-tolerated, some men may experience side effects such as fatigue, skin irritation, and urinary symptoms. Your healthcare provider can help you understand what to expect during treatment and provide guidance on managing any side effects that may arise.

In conclusion, radiation therapy is a valuable treatment option for men with prostate cancer, offering a targeted approach to eliminating cancerous cells and preserving overall prostate health. By working closely with your healthcare provider to develop a personalized treatment plan, you can take proactive steps to address prostate cancer and improve your long-term outcomes. If you have been diagnosed with prostate cancer, consider discussing radiation therapy as a potential treatment option to help you navigate this challenging journey towards better prostate health.

Chapter 7: Coping with a Prostate Health Diagnosis

Emotional Support

Emotional support is a crucial aspect of maintaining overall prostate health. Men often underestimate the impact that emotional well-being can have on their physical health, including the health of their prostate. Stress, anxiety, and depression can all contribute to inflammation and dysfunction within the prostate gland. Therefore, it is essential for men to prioritize their emotional health in order to support the optimal functioning of their prostate.

One key aspect of emotional support for prostate health is seeking out professional help when needed. Men may feel reluctant to talk about their emotions or seek therapy, but it is important to remember that addressing emotional issues can have a positive impact on physical health. Therapists, counselors, and support groups can provide valuable tools and strategies for managing stress, anxiety, and other emotional challenges that may be affecting prostate health.

In addition to professional help, men can also benefit from building a strong support network of friends, family, and loved ones. Having a strong support system can provide emotional stability and encouragement during difficult times. It is important for men to feel comfortable discussing their emotions and seeking help from those they trust.

Physical activity is another important component of emotional support for prostate health. Exercise has been shown to reduce stress, anxiety, and depression, all of which can impact prostate health. Regular physical activity can also help improve mood and overall well-being, leading to a more positive emotional state.

Overall, emotional support plays a critical role in maintaining optimal prostate health. By seeking out professional help, building a strong support network, and incorporating regular physical activity into their routine, men can take proactive steps to support their emotional well-being and promote a healthy prostate. Remember, emotional health is just as important as physical health when it comes to maintaining overall wellness.

Communicating with Loved Ones

Communicating with loved ones about prostate health is an important aspect of maintaining overall well-being. It is essential for men to have open and honest conversations with their family members and partners about any concerns or symptoms related to their prostate health. By keeping loved ones informed, men can receive the support and encouragement they need to prioritize their health and seek appropriate medical care when necessary.

When discussing prostate health with loved ones, it is crucial to approach the topic with sensitivity and empathy. Many men may feel embarrassed or uncomfortable talking about issues such as urinary symptoms or sexual dysfunction. However, by creating a safe and non-judgmental space for open communication, men can feel more comfortable sharing their concerns and seeking advice from their loved ones.

In addition to discussing symptoms and concerns, it is also important for men to communicate with their loved ones about the importance of routine prostate screenings and check-ups. Regular screenings can help detect prostate issues early on, when they are most treatable. By educating their family members about the importance of these screenings, men can receive the support they need to prioritize their health and well-being.

Furthermore, communicating with loved ones about prostate health can also help men navigate treatment options and make informed decisions about their care. By involving their family members in discussions about treatment plans, men can receive valuable input and support as they navigate the complexities of managing prostate health issues. This collaborative approach can help ensure that men feel supported and empowered throughout their treatment journey.

In conclusion, communicating with loved ones about prostate health is a crucial aspect of maintaining overall well-being. By approaching the topic with sensitivity and empathy, men can create a safe space for open and honest conversations with their family members and partners. By keeping loved ones informed about symptoms, concerns, and treatment options, men can receive the support and encouragement they need to prioritize their health and well-being. Ultimately, open communication with loved ones can help men navigate prostate health issues with confidence and empower them to make informed decisions about their care.

Seeking Second Opinions

When faced with a potential prostate health issue, seeking a second opinion can be a crucial step in ensuring you receive the best possible care and treatment. While your primary care physician or urologist may provide valuable insights and recommendations, obtaining a second opinion from another qualified healthcare provider can offer additional perspectives and options for your condition.

One of the main reasons to seek a second opinion is to confirm the initial diagnosis and treatment plan. Prostate health issues can be complex and sometimes difficult to diagnose accurately. By consulting with another healthcare provider, you can ensure that you have received an accurate diagnosis and explore alternative treatment options that may better suit your needs.

Additionally, seeking a second opinion can provide peace of mind and reassurance. Prostate health issues can be stressful and overwhelming, and having another healthcare provider review your case can help alleviate any doubts or uncertainties you may have about your condition. A second opinion can also offer a fresh perspective on your situation and help you make more informed decisions about your treatment plan.

Furthermore, different healthcare providers may have varying areas of expertise and experience with specific prostate health conditions. By seeking a second opinion, you may benefit from the knowledge and insights of a specialist who has dealt with similar cases in the past. This can result in a more personalized and effective treatment plan tailored to your unique needs and circumstances.

In conclusion, seeking a second opinion is a proactive and responsible approach to managing your prostate health. It can provide you with valuable information, peace of mind, and access to a wider range of treatment options. Remember, your health is your most valuable asset, so don't hesitate to seek additional input from another qualified healthcare provider if you have any concerns or questions about your prostate health.

Chapter 8: Preventing Prostate Health Issues

Risk Factors

In order to maintain optimal prostate health, it is important for men to be aware of the various risk factors that can contribute to the development of prostate problems. By understanding these risk factors, men can take proactive steps to reduce their risk and promote overall prostate health.

One of the primary risk factors for prostate problems is age. As men get older, their risk of developing prostate issues increases. It is important for men to be vigilant about their prostate health as they age and to be proactive about getting regular screenings and check-ups.

Another significant risk factor for prostate problems is family history. Men, whose close relatives have had prostate issues, are at a higher risk of developing similar problems themselves. Men with a family history of prostate problems should be especially proactive about monitoring their prostate health and discussing any concerns with their healthcare provider.

Lifestyle factors can also play a significant role in prostate health. Poor diet, lack of exercise, and smoking can all contribute to an increased risk of developing prostate problems. Men should strive to maintain a healthy lifestyle, including a balanced diet and regular exercise, in order to reduce their risk of prostate issues.

Finally, certain medical conditions, such as obesity and diabetes, can also increase the risk of prostate problems. Men who have these conditions should work closely with their healthcare provider to manage their conditions and reduce their risk of developing prostate issues. By being aware of these risk factors and taking proactive steps to address them, men can promote optimal prostate health and reduce their risk of developing prostate problems.

Proactive Steps for Prevention

In order to maintain optimal prostate health, it is essential for men to take proactive steps for prevention. By incorporating certain lifestyle changes and habits into your daily routine, you can greatly reduce your risk of developing prostate issues in the future. Here are some key strategies to consider:

First and foremost, it is crucial to maintain a healthy diet rich in fruits, vegetables, whole grains, and lean proteins. Studies have shown that a diet high in saturated fats and processed foods can contribute to an increased risk of prostate problems. By focusing on a diet that is low in red meat and high in antioxidants, vitamins, and minerals, you can support your prostate health and overall well-being.

Regular exercise is another important factor in preventing prostate issues. Physical activity not only helps to maintain a healthy weight, but it also improves circulation and promotes overall prostate health. Aim for at least 30 minutes of moderate exercise most days of the week, whether it be walking, jogging, swimming, or cycling. Incorporating strength training exercises can also be beneficial for prostate health.

In addition to diet and exercise, it is important for men to schedule regular check-ups with their healthcare provider. Prostate screenings, such as a digital rectal exam or a prostate-specific antigen (PSA) test, can help detect any abnormalities early on. Early detection is key in successfully treating prostate issues, so be sure to discuss the appropriate screening schedule with your doctor based on your age, family history, and risk factors.

Furthermore, it is important to manage stress levels and prioritize mental health. Chronic stress has been linked to inflammation and hormonal imbalances that can negatively impact prostate health. Practice stress-reducing techniques such as meditation, deep breathing exercises, or yoga to help maintain a healthy mind-body connection. Remember, taking care of your mental health is just as important as taking care of your physical health.

By taking proactive steps for prevention, men can significantly reduce their risk of developing prostate issues and promote overall prostate health. By maintaining a healthy diet, regular exercise routine, scheduling regular check-ups, and managing stress levels, you can support your prostate health and well-being for years to come. Remember, it is never too early to start taking care of your prostate health - prevention is key.

Future Developments in Prostate Health

In recent years, there have been significant advancements in the field of prostate health that offer hope for the future of men's health. One exciting development is the use of genetic testing to identify men at higher risk for developing prostate cancer. By understanding their genetic predisposition, men can take proactive measures to reduce their risk and catch the disease in its early stages.

Another promising area of research is the development of new treatments for prostate cancer. Traditional treatments like surgery and radiation therapy can have significant side effects, but emerging therapies such as targeted therapy and immunotherapy show promise in treating the disease with fewer side effects and better outcomes. These treatments could revolutionize the way we approach prostate cancer in the future.

Advancements in imaging technology have also improved our ability to detect and monitor prostate health. MRI scans and other imaging techniques can provide detailed information about the size and location of tumors, allowing for more precise treatment planning. These imaging tools are helping doctors catch prostate cancer earlier and provide more personalized care to their patients.

In the realm of prevention, there is growing evidence that lifestyle factors play a significant role in prostate health. Maintaining a healthy diet, staying physically active, and avoiding tobacco and excessive alcohol consumption can all help reduce the risk of developing prostate cancer. As our understanding of the link between lifestyle and prostate health grows, men can take proactive steps to protect themselves from this disease.

In conclusion, the future of prostate health looks promising, with advancements in genetics, treatment options, imaging technology, and prevention strategies all contributing to better outcomes for men. By staying informed about the latest developments in the field and taking proactive steps to protect their prostate health, men can empower themselves to live longer, healthier lives. The key is to stay educated, stay active, and stay in tune with your body's needs.

Chapter 9: The Role of Mental Health in Prostate Health

Stress and Anxiety

Stress and anxiety are common experiences for many men, but they can have a significant impact on prostate health. When the body is under stress, it releases hormones like cortisol and adrenaline, which can affect the prostate gland and contribute to inflammation and other health issues. Chronic stress can weaken the immune system and make the body more vulnerable to infections and diseases, including prostate cancer.

Men who experience high levels of stress and anxiety may also engage in unhealthy coping mechanisms, such as smoking, excessive drinking, or overeating, which can further exacerbate prostate health problems. Stress can also lead to poor sleep quality, which can disrupt hormonal balance and contribute to prostate issues. It is important for men to find healthy ways to manage stress, such as exercise, meditation, or therapy, in order to protect their prostate health.

Research has shown a strong connection between stress and prostate health, with some studies suggesting that men who experience chronic stress may have a higher risk of developing prostate cancer. Stress can also worsen symptoms of benign prostatic hyperplasia (BPH), a common condition that affects many men as they age. By addressing stress and anxiety through lifestyle changes and stress management techniques, men can potentially reduce their risk of prostate problems and improve their overall health.

In addition to managing stress, it is important for men to prioritize their mental health and seek support when needed. Talking to a therapist or counselor can help men address underlying issues that may be contributing to stress and anxiety. Building a strong support network of friends, family, or a support group can also provide emotional support and help reduce feelings of isolation and loneliness, which can contribute to stress.

Overall, understanding the impact of stress and anxiety on prostate health is crucial for men who want to protect their well-being. By taking proactive steps to manage stress and prioritize mental health, men can reduce their risk of prostate problems and lead healthier, happier lives. It is important for men to recognize the signs of stress and anxiety and seek help when needed in order to maintain optimal prostate health and overall well-being.

Depression and Prostate Health

Depression and prostate health are two interconnected aspects of men's overall well-being that are often overlooked. While depression is typically associated with mental health, it can also have a significant impact on physical health, including prostate health. Research has shown that men suffering from depression are more likely to experience prostate-related issues, such as inflammation and enlargement.

One reason for this correlation is the role that stress plays in both depression and prostate health. Chronic stress can weaken the immune system and increase inflammation in the body, which can contribute to prostate problems. Additionally, men with depression are less likely to engage in healthy behaviors, such as exercise and proper nutrition, which are crucial for maintaining prostate health.

It is essential for men to recognize the connection between depression and prostate health and take steps to address both aspects of their well-being. Seeking treatment for depression, whether through therapy, medication, or lifestyle changes, can help improve mental health and reduce the risk of prostate issues. Additionally, adopting a healthy lifestyle that includes regular exercise, a balanced diet, and stress management techniques can support prostate health and overall well-being.

Men should also prioritize regular screenings and check-ups with their healthcare provider to monitor their prostate health and catch any potential issues early. By taking a proactive approach to both mental and physical health, men can reduce the risk of developing prostate problems and improve their overall quality of life. Remember, taking care of your mental health is just as important as taking care of your physical health when it comes to maintaining prostate health.

Mind-Body Connection

The mind-body connection plays a crucial role in maintaining optimal prostate health. It is well-established that stress, anxiety, and other mental health issues can have a direct impact on physical well-being, including the prostate gland. Research has shown that chronic stress can contribute to inflammation in the body, which in turn can increase the risk of developing prostate conditions such as prostatitis or benign prostatic hyperplasia (BPH). Therefore, it is essential for men to prioritize their mental health in order to support their prostate health.

One way to foster a strong mind-body connection is through regular exercise. Physical activity has been shown to reduce stress levels, improve mood, and boost overall well-being. Exercise also plays a role in maintaining a healthy weight, which is important for prostate health. Men should aim to engage in at least 150 minutes of moderate-intensity exercise per week, such as brisk walking, cycling, or swimming, to support their mental and physical health.

In addition to exercise, mindfulness practices such as meditation, deep breathing, and yoga can help men cultivate a greater awareness of their mental and emotional states. These practices can help reduce stress, improve sleep quality, and enhance overall quality of life. By incorporating mindfulness techniques into their daily routine, men can better manage the stressors that may impact their prostate health.

Another important aspect of the mind-body connection is nutrition. A diet rich in fruits, vegetables, whole grains, and lean proteins can provide the nutrients necessary for optimal prostate health. Certain foods, such as tomatoes, broccoli, and green tea, have been shown to have specific benefits for prostate health. Men should aim to incorporate these foods into their diet regularly to support their prostate health and overall well-being.

In conclusion, the mind-body connection is a critical component of maintaining prostate health. By prioritizing mental health through exercise, mindfulness practices, and a healthy diet, men can support their prostate health and reduce their risk of developing prostate conditions. It is essential for men to take a holistic approach to their health, addressing both mental and physical well-being in order to achieve optimal prostate health.

Chapter 10: Resources for Men's Prostate Health

Support Groups

Support groups can be a valuable resource for men facing prostate health issues. These groups provide a safe space for men to share their experiences, concerns, and emotions with others who are going through similar challenges. By participating in a support group, men can gain valuable insights, advice, and support from fellow members who understand what they are going through.

Support groups can also provide men with access to valuable information and resources that can help them better manage their prostate health. Members can learn about the latest treatments, medications, and lifestyle changes that can improve their overall well-being. Additionally, support groups often invite guest speakers, such as medical professionals or experts in the field of prostate health, to provide valuable insights and guidance to members.

One of the key benefits of joining a support group is the sense of camaraderie and community that it provides. Men often feel isolated and alone when facing prostate health issues, but by joining a support group, they can connect with others who are going through similar experiences. This sense of connection can help men feel less alone and more supported as they navigate their prostate health journey.

Support groups can also provide a platform for men to ask questions, seek advice, and share their concerns in a non-judgmental and understanding environment. Members can offer each other emotional support, practical tips, and encouragement to help one another cope with the challenges of prostate health issues. By participating in a support group, men can gain a sense of empowerment and control over their health and well-being.

In conclusion, support groups can be a valuable resource for men facing prostate health issues. By joining a support group, men can gain access to information, resources, and support that can help them better manage their health. Additionally, support groups provide a sense of community, camaraderie, and empowerment that can help men feel less isolated and more supported as they navigate their prostate health journey. If you are a man dealing with prostate health issues, consider joining a support group to connect with others who understand what you are going through and to gain valuable insights and support.

Educational Materials

In order to maintain optimal prostate health, it is essential for men to educate themselves on the various educational materials available. These resources can provide valuable information on preventive measures, early detection, and treatment options for prostate-related conditions. By taking the time to familiarize oneself with these materials, men can empower themselves to make informed decisions about their health.

One important educational material that men should consider is literature on prostate health. Books such as "Prostate Health Secrets: What Every Man Needs to Know" offer comprehensive information on the prostate gland, common prostate conditions, and strategies for maintaining prostate health. By reading these resources, men can gain a better understanding of the factors that contribute to prostate problems and learn how to take proactive steps to protect their prostate health.

In addition to books, educational videos and online resources can also be valuable tools for men seeking information on prostate health. These materials often feature expert advice from urologists, oncologists, and other healthcare professionals who specialize in prostate care. By watching these videos and reading articles on reputable websites, men can stay informed about the latest developments in prostate health research and treatment.

Another important educational material that men should consider is pamphlets and brochures provided by healthcare providers. These resources often contain practical tips on maintaining prostate health, as well as information on screening tests and treatment options for prostate conditions. By discussing these materials with their doctors, men can receive personalized guidance on how to best protect their prostate health.

In conclusion, educating oneself on prostate health through various materials is crucial for men who want to take control of their well-being. By reading books, watching videos, and discussing information with healthcare providers, men can become better informed about the factors that impact their prostate health and make proactive decisions to protect themselves from prostate-related conditions. Ultimately, investing time in educational materials can empower men to prioritize their prostate health and lead healthier, happier lives.

Healthcare Providers Specializing in Prostate Health

When it comes to prostate health, it is essential to seek care from healthcare providers who specialize in this area. These professionals have a deep understanding of the unique needs and challenges that come with maintaining prostate health. By choosing a healthcare provider who specializes in prostate health, you can ensure that you are receiving the best possible care and treatment for any issues that may arise.

One type of healthcare provider that specializes in prostate health is a urologist. Urologists are medical doctors who have received specialized training in the diagnosis and treatment of conditions affecting the urinary tract and male reproductive system, including the prostate. They are experts in performing procedures such as prostate exams, biopsies, and surgeries, and can provide guidance on managing conditions such as prostate cancer, prostatitis, and benign prostatic hyperplasia.

Another type of healthcare provider that specializes in prostate health is a radiation oncologist. Radiation oncologists are medical doctors who specialize in using radiation therapy to treat cancer. They work closely with urologists and other healthcare providers to develop personalized treatment plans for patients with prostate cancer. Radiation therapy can be an effective treatment option for prostate cancer, either as a primary treatment or in combination with surgery or other therapies.

In addition to urologists and radiation oncologists, there are also nurse practitioners and physician assistants who specialize in prostate health. These advanced practice providers work closely with urologists and other members of the healthcare team to provide comprehensive care for patients with prostate conditions. They can perform prostate exams, order diagnostic tests, prescribe medications, and provide education and support to patients and their families.

Overall, seeking care from healthcare providers who specialize in prostate health is essential for maintaining optimal prostate health and addressing any issues that may arise. By working with these professionals, you can ensure that you are receiving the best possible care and treatment for your prostate condition. Remember to schedule regular check-ups and screenings with your healthcare provider to monitor your prostate health and address any concerns promptly.

Chapter 11: Conclusion

Recap of Key Points

In this subchapter titled "Recap of Key Points," we will review the essential information discussed in the book "Prostate Health Secrets: What Every Man Needs to Know." As men, it is crucial to prioritize our prostate health to prevent the development of serious conditions such as prostate cancer, prostatitis, and benign prostatic hyperplasia (BPH).

First and foremost, regular screenings and check-ups are essential for early detection and treatment of prostate issues. Men should be proactive in discussing any symptoms or concerns with their healthcare provider to ensure timely intervention and management. This includes monitoring PSA levels, undergoing digital rectal exams, and discussing family history of prostate cancer.

Secondly, maintaining a healthy lifestyle through diet and exercise plays a significant role in promoting prostate health. A diet rich in fruits, vegetables, whole grains, and lean proteins can help reduce inflammation and lower the risk of prostate conditions. Regular physical activity, such as brisk walking or cycling, can also improve circulation and reduce the risk of BPH.

Additionally, managing stress and maintaining a healthy weight are crucial factors in prostate health. Chronic stress can contribute to inflammation and hormonal imbalances, which may increase the risk of prostate issues. Maintaining a healthy weight through a balanced diet and regular exercise can help reduce the risk of obesity-related conditions that may impact prostate health.

Lastly, staying informed and educated about prostate health is essential for making informed decisions about screening, treatment options, and lifestyle changes. By staying proactive and taking control of our health, we can reduce the risk of developing prostate conditions and lead a healthier, more fulfilling life. Remember, your prostate health is in your hands, so take charge and prioritize your well-being.

Empowering Men to Take Control of Their Prostate Health

Prostate Health Secrets: What Every Man Needs to Know is dedicated to empowering men to take control of their prostate health. In this subchapter, we will explore the importance of proactive measures in maintaining a healthy prostate and the steps men can take to prevent and manage prostate-related issues. By understanding the significance of prostate health and implementing proactive strategies, men can lead healthier, happier lives.

One of the key ways to empower men in taking control of their prostate health is through education. Many men are unaware of the importance of regular prostate screenings and the potential risks associated with prostate issues. By educating themselves on the topic, men can make informed decisions about their health and take proactive steps to prevent and manage prostate-related conditions.

In addition to education, self-care practices play a crucial role in maintaining prostate health. This includes adopting a healthy diet, engaging in regular physical activity, and avoiding habits that can negatively impact prostate health, such as smoking and excessive alcohol consumption. By prioritizing self-care and making healthy lifestyle choices, men can significantly reduce their risk of developing prostate issues.

Regular prostate screenings are another essential aspect of empowering men to take control of their prostate health. Early detection of prostate issues is key to successful treatment and management. Men should work with their healthcare providers to establish a screening schedule that aligns with their age and risk factors, ensuring that any potential issues are identified and addressed promptly.

By combining education, self-care practices, and regular screenings, men can proactively manage their prostate health and reduce their risk of developing prostate-related conditions. Empowering men to take control of their prostate health is essential for promoting overall well-being and longevity. By taking proactive steps and prioritizing their health, men can enjoy a higher quality of life and reduce the likelihood of experiencing prostate-related issues in the future.

Looking Ahead: The Future of Prostate Health

As men, it is important to prioritize our prostate health in order to maintain overall well-being and quality of life. Looking ahead, the future of prostate health holds promising advancements in both prevention and treatment options. By staying informed and proactive about our health, we can take steps to reduce the risk of developing prostate-related conditions and ensure early detection if necessary.

One of the key areas of focus for the future of prostate health is early detection through advanced screening technologies. With the development of more accurate and sensitive tests, such as the prostate-specific antigen (PSA) test and MRI imaging, doctors can detect prostate cancer at earlier stages when it is more easily treatable. By staying up to date on the latest screening recommendations and discussing them with our healthcare providers, we can take proactive steps to monitor our prostate health and catch any potential issues early on.

In addition to advancements in early detection, the future of prostate health also holds promising developments in treatment options. From minimally invasive surgical techniques to targeted radiation therapies, men facing prostate cancer have more choices than ever before when it comes to managing their condition. By staying informed about the latest treatment options and discussing them with our healthcare team, we can make more informed decisions about our prostate health and overall well-being.

Furthermore, the future of prostate health also includes a greater emphasis on lifestyle factors that can impact prostate health. By maintaining a healthy diet rich in fruits, vegetables, and whole grains, staying active, and avoiding tobacco and excessive alcohol consumption, men can reduce their risk of developing prostate-related conditions. Additionally, staying at a healthy weight and managing stress levels can also play a role in promoting prostate health and overall wellness.

In conclusion, looking ahead at the future of prostate health offers hope for improved detection, treatment, and prevention options for men. By staying informed, proactive, and engaged in our healthcare, we can take control of our prostate health and make choices that support our overall well-being. Let us commit to prioritizing our prostate health and taking the necessary steps to ensure a healthy future for ourselves.

9 798334 743625